Cystic fibrosis gene

Full details on how genetic can affect the lungs and how you can get it treated

Dr Joe smith

Contents

Chapter1

Introduction to cystic fibrosis

Cystic fibrosis (CF) is a genetic disorder that affects the lungs, pancreas, and other organs. It is a life-threatening condition that primarily affects the respiratory and digestive systems, leading to progressive lung damage, difficulty breathing, and malnutrition. CF is a relatively rare disease, with approximately 30,000 people living with the condition in the United States and about 70,000 people worldwide. The first recorded case of cystic fibrosis was in 1938, when Dr. Dorothy Anderson identified it as a distinct medical condition. However, it was not until the 1950s that researchers began to understand the cause of CF – a faulty gene known as the cystic fibrosis transmembrane conductance regulator (CFTR). This gene is responsible for creating a protein that regulates the movement of salt and water in and out of cells. In a person with CF, this protein does not function properly, causing a build-up of thick, sticky mucus in the lungs and other organs. The mucus traps bacteria and other foreign particles, leading to frequent respiratory infections and difficulty breathing. In the pancreas, the mucus obstructs the normal function of the organ, preventing the release of enzymes needed for proper digestion and absorption of nutrients. This results in malnutrition and growth issues in individuals with CF. CF is an autosomal recessive disorder, meaning that both parents must carry a mutated copy of the CFTR gene for a child to inherit the condition. If both parents are carriers, there is a 25% chance of having a child with CF. If only one parent carries the gene, the child will not have the disease but may inherit the gene and pass it on to their children. Fortunately, there are now tests available to identify carriers of the gene, allowing couples to make informed decisions about having children. Symptoms of CF can vary in severity and may present differently in each individual. However, some of the common symptoms include frequent respiratory infections, difficulty breathing, coughing, wheezing, and frequent production of thick, sticky mucus. In the digestive system, symptoms may include malnutrition, poor weight gain, and bulky, greasy stools. These symptoms often appear in childhood, and the severity of the condition tends to worsen over time. Due to the complex nature of the disease, CF requires lifelong management and treatment. There is currently no cure for CF, but advances in medical research and treatments have significantly improved the quality and length of life for individuals with the condition. The main goal of treatment is to prevent and manage complications, alleviate symptoms, and improve the overall function of organs affected by the disease. One of the primary treatment options for CF is daily airway clearance techniques, which help loosen and remove mucus from the lungs, allowing for easier breathing. This may include postural drainage, chest percussion, and the use of a positive expiratory pressure (PEP) device. Medications such as antibiotics, bronchodilators, and mucolytics may also be prescribed to help prevent and treat respiratory infections and improve lung function. Individuals with CF also require a specialized diet due to the inability to properly digest and absorb nutrients. A high-calorie and high-fat diet, along with pancreatic enzyme replacement therapy, is often recommended to help maintain a healthy weight and prevent malnutrition. In severe cases, a feeding tube or other nutritional support may be necessary. Another crucial aspect of CF treatment is the management of chronic lung infections. People with CF are at a higher risk of developing respiratory infections due to the build-up of mucus in their lungs. These infections can be life-threatening and require aggressive antibiotic treatment. In some cases, individuals with CF may need to be hospitalized for intravenous (IV) antibiotic therapy. Along with medical treatment, individuals with CF also require regular check-ups and monitoring by a team of healthcare professionals specialized in treating the condition. This may include pulmonologists, respiratory therapists, dietitians, and physical therapists. The frequency of check-ups and the type of treatment may vary depending on the individual's age and the severity of their condition. Despite the challenges and complexities of living with CF, many people with the condition are living productive and fulfilling lives. Advances in medical research and treatments have significantly improved the life expectancy of individuals with CF, with many now living into their 40s, 50s, and beyond. However, CF is still a progressive and life-threatening disease that requires continuous care and management for the best possible outcome. In conclusion, cystic fibrosis is a genetic disorder that affects the lungs, pancreas, and other organs, leading to progressive lung damage, difficulty breathing, and malnutrition. It is caused by a faulty gene known as the CFTR gene, and its symptoms typically appear in childhood. While there is no cure for CF, proper management and treatment can improve the quality of life for individuals with the condition. With ongoing research and advancements in medical technology, it is hoped that one day a cure for cystic fibrosis will be found.

chapter2

cystic fibrosistreatment

While there is no cure for cystic fibrosis, there are various treatments available that can help manage the symptoms and improve the quality of life for those living with this condition. In this essay, we will discuss the different treatment options for cystic fibrosis. 1. Airway Clearance Techniques: The most common and crucial aspect of cystic fibrosis treatment is airway clearance techniques. These techniques help to remove the thick and sticky mucus from the airways, thus reducing the risk of lung infections and improving lung function. There are various airway clearance techniques, such as vibration and percussion, chest physiotherapy, and positive expiratory pressure devices. These techniques can be performed at home or with the help of a respiratory therapist. 2. Medications: There are several medications used for the treatment of cystic fibrosis. These medications aim to decrease mucus production, fight lung infections, and improve lung function. Some common medications include bronchodilators, which help to open up the airways, antibiotics to fight lung infections, and mucolytic agents to reduce mucus production. In addition, some patients may also need pancreatic enzymes to aid in digestion and vitamin supplements to prevent nutritional deficiencies. 3. Lung Transplant: In severe cases of cystic fibrosis, where the lungs are severely damaged, a lung transplant may be considered. A lung transplant involves replacing the diseased lung with a healthy one from a donor. This procedure can significantly improve the quality of life for the patient. However, it is a complex and risky surgery, and not all patients are suitable candidates for it.

4. Gene Therapy: Gene therapy is a relatively new approach towards treating cystic fibrosis. It involves correcting the genetic defect responsible for the condition. This therapy attempts to replace the faulty gene with a healthy one, thus improving the function of the cells and reducing the severity of symptoms. While gene therapy shows promising results, it is still in the early stages of development, and further

research is needed before it can be widely used as a treatment for cystic fibrosis. 5. Nutritional Therapy: Cystic fibrosis can affect the digestive system, leading to malabsorption of vital nutrients. Therefore, patients with this condition need a high-calorie, high-protein diet to maintain their weight and prevent malnutrition. They may also require vitamin and mineral supplements to ensure they receive adequate nutrition. In some cases, a feeding tube may be inserted to deliver nutrients directly to the stomach, especially in patients with severe lung disease. 6. Physical Activity: Regular physical activity is an essential part of managing cystic fibrosis. It can help improve lung function, reduce the amount of mucus in the airways, and strengthen the muscles involved in breathing. However, it is essential to consult a healthcare professional before engaging in physical activity, as the intensity and type of exercise may vary depending on the severity of the condition and the individual's abilities.

7. Psychological Support: Living with a chronic illness like cystic fibrosis can take a toll on a person both physically and emotionally. Hence, it is crucial to provide psychological support to patients and their families. This support can come in the form of counseling, joining support groups, or talking to a therapist. These sessions can help patients and their families understand

and cope with the challenges of living with cystic fibrosis.

chapter3

cystic fibrosis symptoms

The most common and significant symptom of cystic fibrosis is respiratory issues. The thick and sticky mucus that builds up in the lungs makes it difficult to breathe, leading to frequent lung infections and inflammation. These infections can cause coughing, wheezing, and shortness of breath, primarily during physical activity. As the disease progresses, the lungs become more damaged, and breathing difficulties become more severe. Chronic bronchitis and bronchiectasis (damaged airways) are also common respiratory complications of cystic fibrosis. Digestive problems are another hallmark symptom of cystic fibrosis. The thick mucus can block the ducts of the pancreas, preventing digestive enzymes from reaching the small intestine. As a result, people with CF may have difficulty digesting and absorbing fats, proteins, and vitamins in their diet. This can lead to malnutrition and vitamin deficiencies, particularly in vitamins A, D, E, and K. These deficiencies can cause a range of symptoms, including poor growth and weight gain, frequent stools, abdominal pain, and bloating. The thick mucus can also cause blockages in the bile ducts, leading to liver damage and inflammation. Over time, this can cause scarring and permanent damage to the liver, leading to liver failure or cirrhosis. Liver disease is more common in adults with CF, and symptoms may include jaundice (yellowing of the skin and eyes), fatigue, and abdominal pain. Another significant symptom of cystic fibrosis is sweat gland dysfunction. People with CF have significantly higher levels of salt in their sweat, resulting in unusually salty skin. This is one of the most common signs of the disease and can help doctors in making a diagnosis. This excessive salt in the sweat can also lead to dehydration and electrolyte imbalances, causing fatigue, weakness, and heat exhaustion. The effects of cystic fibrosis on the immune system can also lead to a range of symptoms. The thick mucus in the lungs provides a breeding ground for bacteria, resulting in frequent infections. These infections can cause coughing up mucus, wheezing, shortness of breath, chest pain, and fatigue. As the bacteria become more resistant to antibiotics, they can cause severe and even life-threatening lung infections, such as pneumonia and bronchitis. Cystic fibrosis can also affect the reproductive system, particularly in men. Due to the thick mucus blocking the vas deferens (a tube that carries sperm), males with CF may experience fertility problems and be unable to father children naturally. In females, the reproductive mucus may also be affected, making it difficult for them to conceive. Apart from the physical symptoms, cystic fibrosis can also affect mental health. The constant struggle with symptoms, hospitalizations, and a shortened life expectancy can cause emotional distress, anxiety, depression, and stress in individuals with CF. Furthermore, the financial burden of treatments, medications, and hospital stays can also lead to additional stress and anxiety for both the individual with CF and their family. Early diagnosis and treatment play a crucial role in managing the symptoms of cystic fibrosis effectively. The majority of individuals with CF are diagnosed in childhood, often after symptoms are apparent, or a newborn screening test shows an abnormality. However, in some cases, people may not be diagnosed until later in life, particularly if their symptoms are mild. There is currently no cure for cystic fibrosis, and treatment focuses on managing symptoms, preventing complications, and improving quality of life. This includes a combination of medications, therapies, and lifestyle modifications. Inhaled treatments are used to help clear the mucus from the lungs and prevent infections, while digestive enzyme supplements can aid in the absorption of nutrients. Antibiotics may also be prescribed to treat bacterial infections, and treatments to thin the mucus may be beneficial. Regular exercise and a healthy diet are essential in managing cystic fibrosis symptoms. Exercise can improve lung function, help clear mucus from airways, and improve overall fitness and strength. A high-calorie, high-fat diet is crucial for people with CF to maintain a healthy weight and receive adequate nutrition. In recent years, there have been significant advancements in the treatment of cystic fibrosis, including new medications that target specific mutations of the CF gene and therapies that help improve lung function. However, living with cystic fibrosis still presents many challenges, and individuals with the condition require ongoing support and medical care.

cystic fibrosis causes

The CFTR gene contains instructions for making the CFTR protein, which is found on the surface of cells in many organs, including the lungs, pancreas, liver, and intestines. In healthy individuals, this protein acts as a channel, allowing salts and fluids to move in and out of cells. The movement of these substances is essential for maintaining a healthy balance of fluids and electrolytes in the body. However, in people with CF, the CFTR gene is defective and does not produce the CFTR protein or produces a faulty version of it. This results in several problems, such as thick mucus production and improper regulation of salt and fluid movement in the body. One of the main causes of CF is inheriting a mutated CFTR gene from both parents. This is known as autosomal recessive inheritance, meaning that both copies of the gene must be mutated for the disease to develop. If the child inherits one copy of the mutated gene from one parent and a normal gene from the other, they will be a carrier of the disease but will not have CF. However, if two carriers have a child, there is a 25% chance that the child will inherit two copies of the mutated gene and develop CF. The most common mutation in the CFTR gene is known as Delta F508 and is responsible for about 70% of CF cases worldwide. Other less common mutations in the CFTR gene can also cause CF, but their prevalence varies among different populations. These mutations can lead to a range of CF symptoms, severity, and complications. Another cause of CF can be attributed to a phenomenon known as mosaicism. This occurs when a person has two different cells in their body, one with a normal copy of the

CFTR gene and the other with a mutated one. In this case, the person may not develop CF or may have a milder form of the disease. Mosaicism occurs randomly during early fetal development and is extremely rare. Apart from genetic causes, environmental factors can also contribute to the development and severity of CF. Exposure to certain toxic substances, such as cigarette smoke, can increase the risk of developing CF or worsen symptoms in people with the disease. Additionally, people with CF have a compromised immune system, making them more susceptible to infections that can further damage their lungs and other organs. Lung infections are a major complication of CF and are the primary cause of morbidity and mortality in people with this disease. The thick mucus in the lungs provides an ideal environment for bacteria to grow, leading to frequent and severe respiratory infections. The most common bacteria that cause lung infections in people with CF are Staphylococcus aureus, Pseudomonas aeruginosa, and Haemophilus influenzae. The mucus buildup in the lungs also impairs the ability to clear out these infections, making it harder to get rid of them. Over time, these repeated infections cause irreversible damage to the lung tissue, leading to lung scarring, bronchiectasis, and eventually respiratory failure. In addition to lung infections, people with CF also have increased mucus production in the pancreas, which can lead to pancreatic insufficiency. This means that the pancreas cannot produce enough enzymes to help break down and absorb nutrients from food. As a result, people with CF may have difficulty gaining weight or may experience malnutrition. This can also lead to problems with the gastrointestinal tract, such as intestinal obstruction, GERD (gastroesophageal reflux disease), and rectal prolapse. Moreover, the thick mucus in the pancreas can also block the ducts that carry digestive enzymes to the small intestine, causing inflammation and scarring of the pancreas. This condition is known as pancreatitis and can lead to severe abdominal pain, diarrhea, and malabsorption of nutrients. Another common symptom of CF is salty-tasting skin. People with CF lose more salt in their sweat than those without the condition. This can lead to electrolyte imbalances and dehydration, especially during hot weather or physical activity.

chapter4

cystic fibrosis gene

The CFTR gene is located on the long arm of chromosome 7 and contains 27 exons that code for a 1,480 amino acid protein. Over 2000 different mutations have been identified in this gene, with the most common one being the deltaF508 mutation, which causes about 70% of all cystic fibrosis cases. This mutation results in a deletion of three nucleotides in the CFTR gene, leading to the deletion of a single amino acid (phenylalanine) in the protein. This small change in the protein structure disrupts its function and leads to the characteristic symptoms of cystic fibrosis. Cystic fibrosis is an autosomal recessive disorder, which means that a person needs to inherit two copies of the mutated gene (one from each parent) to develop the disease. Individuals who have only one copy of the mutated gene are known as carriers and do not usually have any symptoms of the disorder. One of the major consequences of cystic fibrosis is the thick, sticky mucus that accumulates in the lungs. This mucus traps bacteria, viruses, and other microorganisms, leading to frequent lung infections and inflammation. As a result, individuals with cystic fibrosis have a reduced ability to breathe, and over time, this can lead to permanent lung damage and respiratory failure. The mucus also affects the function of the pancreas and inhibits the release of enzymes that help break down food, leading to malnutrition and poor growth. The severity and frequency of symptoms in cystic fibrosis vary from person to person and largely depend on the type of CFTR gene mutation an individual has inherited. Some mutations are associated with milder symptoms, while others can be life-threatening. In addition to lung and digestive problems, cystic fibrosis can also affect other organs, such as the liver, spleen, and reproductive system. Diagnosis of cystic fibrosis involves a series of tests, including a sweat test, which measures the amount of salt (chloride) in the sweat. People with cystic fibrosis have unusually high levels of salt in their sweat due to the malfunctioning proteins that regulate salt transport. Genetic testing can also be done to confirm the presence of mutations in the CFTR gene. Unfortunately, there is currently no cure for cystic fibrosis, and treatment mainly focuses on managing the symptoms and preventing complications. This may involve medications to thin the mucus and improve lung function, inhalers to open up the airways, and antibiotics to treat infections. In some cases, lung transplantation or pancreatic enzyme replacement therapy may be necessary. Advances in genetic research have led to the development of new treatments for cystic fibrosis, particularly targeted therapies that can correct specific mutations in the CFTR gene. These treatments are known as CFTR modulators and have shown promising results in improving lung function and reducing hospitalizations in people with cystic fibrosis. However, they are currently only available for a small percentage of individuals with specific mutations, and more research is needed in this area. Cystic fibrosis can have a significant impact on a person's life, and managing the disease can be challenging, both physically and emotionally. Individuals with cystic fibrosis require regular medical monitoring and treatment, which can be time-consuming and expensive. The disease can also affect the mental health of patients, as they often face physical limitations and have to deal with multiple hospitalizations and treatments. Despite these challenges, people with cystic fibrosis can live relatively healthy and fulfilling lives, thanks to advances in medical care. The average lifespan of individuals with cystic fibrosis has significantly improved over the years, with the current median age of survival being approximately 47 years. However, the severity and progression of the disease can vary greatly, and some individuals may have a significantly shorter lifespan. In addition to medical treatments, lifestyle modifications, such as a healthy diet and regular exercise, can also help manage the symptoms and improve the overall quality of life for people with cystic fibrosis. Physical therapy and breathing exercises can also help improve lung function and prevent respiratory complications.

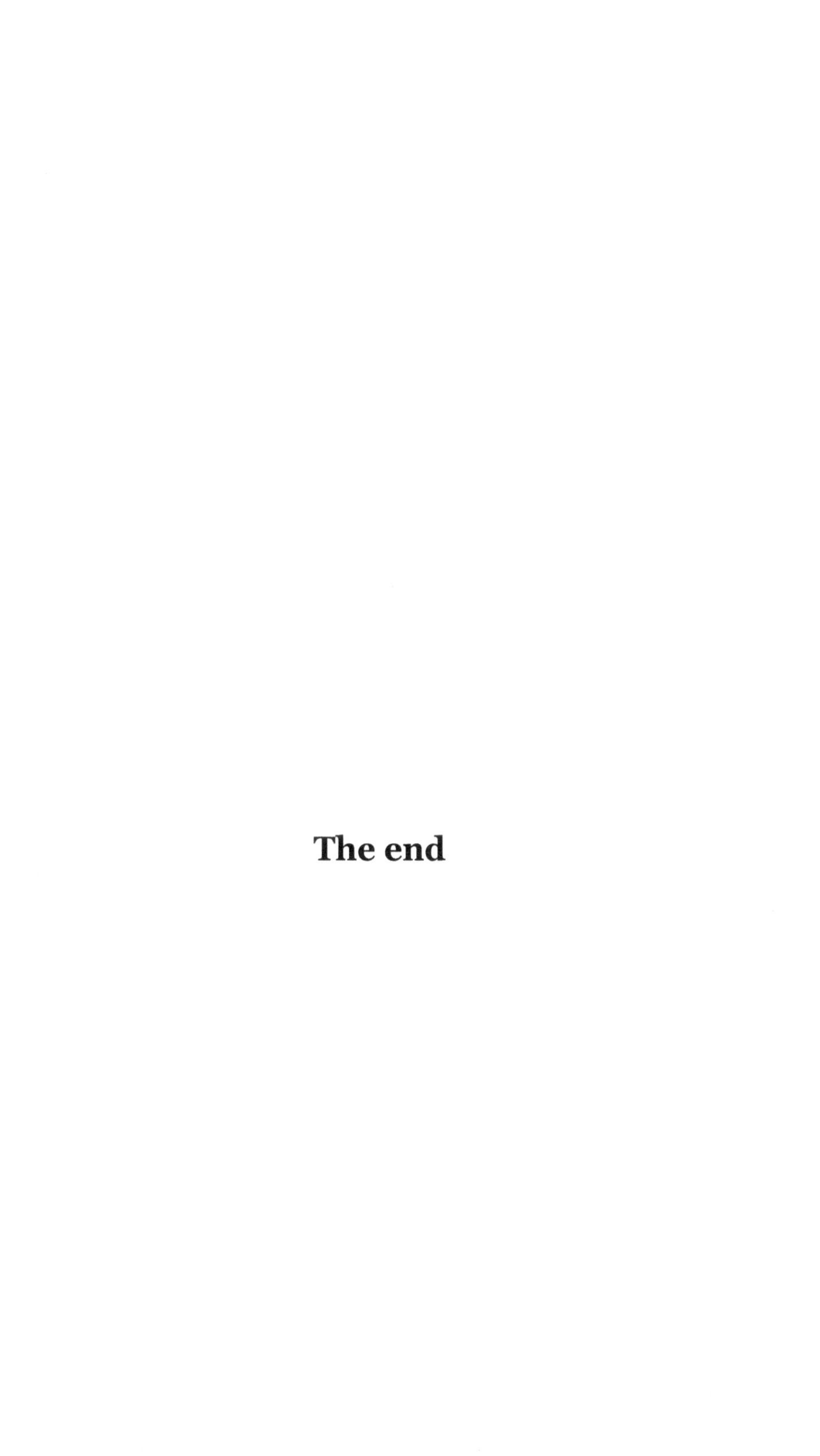

The end